CELIAC DISEASE COOKBOOK FOR SENIORS

Nutritious, Delicious and Easy-to-Make Gluten-Free Recipes for Healthy and Vibrant Life

Sonia Emmason

CHAPTER 1

INTRODUCTION TO CELIAC DISEASE DIET FOR SENIORS

Celiac disease is an autoimmune disorder that affects people of all ages, but it is particularly common in seniors. This condition causes the immune system to react negatively to gluten, a protein found in wheat, barley, and rye. The reaction damages the lining of the small intestine, which can lead to a range of symptoms, including abdominal pain, diarrhea, fatigue, weight loss, and anemia. The only known treatment for celiac disease is a strict gluten-free diet.

The good news is that there are plenty of delicious and healthy gluten-free foods that seniors can enjoy as part of a balanced diet. With a little bit of knowledge and planning, seniors with celiac disease can still enjoy tasty and satisfying meals that meet their nutritional needs.

One of the key challenges of following a gluten-free diet is learning how to identify and avoid gluten-containing foods.

This can be particularly challenging for seniors who may have limited mobility or access to specialty foods. However, with the help of a celiac disease dietitian or nutritionist, seniors can learn how to navigate food labels, identify safe gluten-free products, and plan healthy meals that meet their dietary needs.

Another important aspect of a celiac disease diet for seniors is ensuring that they are getting all the nutrients they need. Gluten-free diets can be low in certain nutrients, including fiber, iron, calcium, and vitamin D. Seniors may also have additional nutritional needs due to age-related changes in their bodies. Working with a registered dietitian can help seniors identify potential nutrient deficiencies and find ways to incorporate nutrient-rich foods into their diets.

In addition to dietary considerations, seniors with celiac disease may also need to be mindful of social situations that involve food. Eating out, attending parties, or visiting friends and family can all present challenges for seniors with celiac disease.

However, with some planning and communication, it is possible to enjoy social events without compromising dietary needs. Seniors can bring their own gluten-free dishes to potlucks or ask for gluten-free options at restaurants. Friends and family members can also be educated about the dietary restrictions associated with celiac disease, so they can provide appropriate options when hosting seniors with celiac disease.

Ultimately, following a celiac disease diet can be a challenging but rewarding experience for seniors. By making a commitment to a gluten-free lifestyle and working with healthcare professionals to develop a personalized nutrition plan, seniors with celiac disease can enjoy a healthy and vibrant life. Whether cooking at home, dining out, or socializing with friends and family, seniors can find ways to incorporate delicious and nutritious gluten-free foods into their diets and live life to the fullest.

CHAPTER 2

2.1 WHAT IS CELIAC DISEASE?

Celiac disease is an autoimmune disorder that affects the small intestine. It is caused by a reaction to gluten, a protein found in wheat, barley, and rye. When someone with celiac disease consumes gluten, their immune system reacts negatively, causing damage to the lining of the small intestine. This damage can lead to a range of symptoms, including abdominal pain, bloating, diarrhea, constipation, weight loss, fatigue, and anemia. Over time, the damage to the small intestine can also lead to malnutrition, which can cause additional health problems.

Celiac disease is a genetic condition, which means that it tends to run in families. It is estimated that about 1 in 100 people worldwide have celiac disease, though many cases go undiagnosed or are misdiagnosed as other conditions. The only known treatment for celiac disease is a strict gluten-free diet. By avoiding gluten-containing foods, people with celiac disease can manage their symptoms and prevent further damage to their small intestine.

Celiac disease symptoms in seniors can be similar to those experienced by younger adults, but there are some differences. Seniors may be more likely to have atypical symptoms, which can make it harder to diagnose celiac disease. Here are some of the common symptoms of celiac disease in seniors:

1. **Digestive problems:** Seniors with celiac disease may experience symptoms such as abdominal pain, bloating, gas, diarrhea, and constipation. These symptoms can be particularly disruptive to seniors' lives, as they can interfere with daily activities and reduce quality of life.

2. **Anemia:** Celiac disease can cause anemia, a condition in which the body does not have enough red blood cells to carry oxygen to the body's tissues. Anemia can cause fatigue, weakness, and shortness of breath, and it can be particularly

dangerous for seniors who may already have other health issues.

3. **Osteoporosis:** Celiac disease can lead to bone loss and osteoporosis, a condition in which bones become weak and brittle. Seniors with celiac disease may be more susceptible to fractures and other bone-related injuries.

4. **Neurological symptoms:** In some cases, celiac disease can cause neurological symptoms, such as headache, numbness or tingling in the hands and feet, and difficulty with balance and coordination.

5. **Skin rash:** Some seniors with celiac disease may develop a skin rash called dermatitis herpetiformis. This rash is characterized by itchy, blistering bumps that usually appear on the elbows, knees, buttocks, and scalp.

It is important to note that not all seniors with celiac disease will experience these symptoms, and some may have no symptoms at all. If you are a senior and you suspect you may have celiac disease, it is important to talk to your doctor about getting tested.

Early diagnosis and treatment can help prevent further health complications and improve quality of life.

2.3 DIAGNOSING CELIAC DISEASE

Celiac disease is an autoimmune disorder that affects the small intestine. It occurs when the body's immune system responds to gluten, a protein found in wheat, barley, and rye, by attacking the lining of the small intestine. This results in damage to the intestinal lining and prevents the body from absorbing nutrients properly.

Diagnosing celiac disease typically involves a combination of blood tests, genetic testing, and a biopsy of the small intestine.

1. **Blood tests:** Blood tests can measure the levels of certain antibodies in your blood. People with celiac disease have higher levels of antibodies called tissue transglutaminase (tTG) and endomysial antibodies (EMA). If these antibodies are elevated, it is an indication that the immune system is reacting to gluten.

2. **Genetic testing:** A simple blood test can determine if you carry the genes associated with celiac disease. However, having these genes alone does not necessarily mean you have celiac disease, as many people with these genes do not develop the condition.

3. **Biopsy:** A biopsy of the small intestine is considered the gold standard for diagnosing celiac disease. During a biopsy, a small piece of tissue is removed from the lining of the small intestine and examined under a microscope for damage to the villi, which are tiny finger-like projections that help absorb nutrients. If the villi are flattened, it is a sign of celiac disease.

It is important to continue consuming gluten until all testing is completed. Eliminating gluten from the diet before testing can lead to false negative results. If celiac disease is diagnosed, the only effective treatment is a lifelong gluten-free diet. A dietitian or doctor can provide guidance on how to follow a gluten-free diet and ensure you are getting all the nutrients your body needs.

CHAPTER 3

MANAGING CELIAC DISEASE

Managing celiac disease in seniors requires a multifaceted approach that addresses both the physical and emotional aspects of the condition. Here are some tips for managing celiac disease in seniors:

1. **Follow a strict gluten-free diet:** The only effective treatment for celiac disease is a lifelong gluten-free diet. This means avoiding all sources of gluten, including wheat, barley, and rye. Seniors may need help from family members or caregivers to ensure that their diet is free of gluten.

2. **Monitor for nutrient deficiencies:** Celiac disease can cause malabsorption of nutrients, which can lead to deficiencies in vitamins and minerals. Seniors may be at higher risk for nutrient deficiencies due to factors such as reduced appetite, decreased absorption, and medication interactions. Regular blood tests can help identify any deficiencies, and a registered

dietitian can help develop a personalized plan to address them.

3. **Manage other health conditions:** Seniors with celiac disease may have other health conditions that require management, such as osteoporosis, diabetes, or high blood pressure. It is important to work with healthcare providers to develop a comprehensive plan for managing all health conditions.

4. **Stay socially connected:** Seniors with celiac disease may feel isolated or left out of social events that involve food. Encourage seniors to stay socially connected and to communicate their dietary needs to family members, friends, and caregivers. There are also support groups and online communities for people with celiac disease that can provide a sense of community and connection.

5. **Address mental health concerns:** Seniors with celiac disease may experience anxiety, depression, or other mental health concerns related to the challenges of managing a strict

gluten-free diet. It is important to address these concerns and provide support as needed, such as through therapy or counseling.

Overall, managing celiac disease in seniors requires a holistic approach that addresses both the physical and emotional aspects of the condition. With proper management, seniors with celiac disease can maintain good health and quality of life.

CHAPTER 4

GLUTEN-FREE DIET GUIDELINES

A gluten-free diet is a diet that excludes gluten, a protein found in wheat, barley, and rye. It is essential for people with celiac disease, gluten intolerance, or gluten sensitivity. Here are some guidelines to follow if you're on a gluten-free diet:

1. Avoid all foods that contain wheat, barley, and rye. This includes all products made with these grains, such as bread, pasta, cereals, crackers, and baked goods.

2. Choose gluten-free grains and starches. This includes rice, corn, quinoa, buckwheat, amaranth, and potatoes. Be sure to check labels to ensure that the products are truly gluten-free.

3. Be aware of hidden sources of gluten. Gluten can be found in many processed foods, such as canned soups, sauces, and dressings. It can also be found in some medications, vitamins, and supplements. Always check the labels for gluten-containing ingredients.

4. Avoid cross-contamination. Even trace amounts of gluten can be harmful to people with celiac disease or gluten intolerance. Use separate cooking utensils, cutting boards, and toasters for gluten-free foods.

5. Choose gluten-free alternatives for foods you normally eat. Many gluten-free products are available, such as bread, pasta, and crackers. However, some of these products may contain high amounts of sugar, salt, and fat. Be sure to read the labels and choose products that are healthy and nutrient-dense.

6. Focus on whole, unprocessed foods. Fresh fruits, vegetables, meats, and fish are naturally gluten-free and provide important nutrients for overall health.

7. Work with a registered dietitian. A registered dietitian can help you plan a balanced gluten-free diet and ensure that you're getting all the nutrients you need.

Remember that a gluten-free diet is not a weight-loss diet.

It's a medical necessity for people with celiac disease or gluten intolerance. Be sure to follow these guidelines to ensure that you're maintaining a healthy and balanced diet while avoiding gluten.

CHAPTER 5

PANTRY ESSENTIALS FOR A GLUTEN-FREE DIET

If you're following a gluten-free diet, it's important to have a well-stocked pantry of gluten-free essentials to help you prepare meals and snacks. Here are some pantry staples to keep on hand:

1. **Gluten-free flour:** This can be used as a substitute for wheat flour in recipes. Popular gluten-free flours include rice flour, almond flour, coconut flour, and chickpea flour.

2. **Gluten-free pasta:** There are many types of gluten-free pasta available, including those made from rice, corn, quinoa, and lentils.

3. **Gluten-free grains:** Stock up on gluten-free grains like rice, quinoa, millet, buckwheat, and amaranth. These can be used as a base for meals, as a side dish, or in salads.

4. **Nuts and seeds:** Nuts and seeds are great for snacking, as well as adding flavor and nutrition to meals. Almonds, cashews, walnuts, chia seeds, and flax seeds are all good choices.

5. **Canned beans and lentils:** Canned beans and lentils are a quick and easy source of protein, fiber, and other nutrients. Choose varieties that are labeled as gluten-free.

6. **Gluten-free bread or wraps:** Look for gluten-free bread or wraps made from alternative grains like rice, quinoa, or corn.

7. **Gluten-free oats:** If you're sensitive to gluten, make sure to choose oats that are labeled as gluten-free to avoid cross-contamination.

8. **Gluten-free crackers and chips:** These are great for snacking, and can be used in place of bread for dips and spreads.

9. **Canned tomatoes and tomato sauce:** Tomatoes are a versatile ingredient that can be used in a variety of dishes. Make sure to choose varieties that are labeled as gluten-free.

10. **Spices and seasonings:** Keep a variety of gluten-free spices and seasonings on hand to add flavor to your meals.

Remember to always check labels carefully when buying packaged or processed foods to ensure that they are gluten-free. Additionally, if you have any questions or concerns about your gluten-free diet, speak with a registered dietitian for personalized advice and guidance.

CHAPTER 6

6.0 HEALTHY AND DELICIOUS CELIAC DISEASE RECIPES FOR SENIORS

6.1 BREAKFAST RECIPES

1. Oats and Quinoa Porridge (15 minutes)

Ingredients:

- ½ cup gluten-free rolled oats

- ¼ cup quinoa flakes

- 2 cups water

- ¼ teaspoon ground cinnamon

- 1 tablespoon honey

- ¼ cup chopped nuts (optional)

Instructions:

1. In a medium saucepan, combine the oats, quinoa flakes, and water.

2. Bring to a boil, then reduce the heat and simmer for 10 minutes, stirring occasionally.

3. Add the cinnamon and honey, and stir to combine.

4. Serve in a bowl and top with chopped nuts, if desired.

Ingredients:

- 4 medium apples, cored and sliced

- 2 tablespoons coconut oil, melted

- 2 tablespoons honey

- 2 tablespoons chopped walnuts

- 2 tablespoons chopped almonds

- 2 tablespoons unsweetened shredded coconut

- 1 teaspoon ground cinnamon

Instructions:

1. Preheat the oven to 350°F.

2. Place the apples in a shallow baking dish.

3. In a small bowl, combine the coconut oil, honey, walnuts, almonds, coconut, and cinnamon.

4. Pour the mixture over the apples and toss to coat.

5. Bake for 20 minutes, stirring once or twice during baking.

Ingredients:

- 6 large eggs

- 1 cup chopped cooked vegetables (e.g., bell peppers, onions, mushrooms)

- 1 cup chopped cooked sausage or bacon

- 2 tablespoons chopped fresh herbs (e.g., parsley, chives, basil)

- Salt and pepper to taste

Instructions:

1. Preheat the oven to 350°F.

2. Grease a 12-cup muffin tin with cooking spray.

3. In a large bowl, whisk together the eggs, vegetables, sausage or bacon, herbs, salt, and pepper.

4. Divide the mixture among the muffin cups.

5. Bake for 15-20 minutes, or until the muffins are cooked through and the edges are golden brown.

Ingredients:

- 1 cup unsweetened almond milk

- ¼ cup chia seeds

- 1 teaspoon honey

- ¼ teaspoon ground cinnamon

- ¼ cup chopped nuts (optional)

Instructions:

1. In a medium bowl, combine the almond milk, chia seeds, honey, and cinnamon.

2. Stir to combine and let sit for 5 minutes.

3. Stir again and let sit for another 5 minutes.

4. Transfer the mixture to an airtight container and chill in the refrigerator overnight.

5. Serve chilled and top with chopped nuts, if desired.

Ingredients:

- 1 ripe banana, peeled and sliced

- ½ cup unsweetened almond milk

- 2 tablespoons almond butter

- 1 teaspoon ground flaxseed

- ½ teaspoon ground cinnamon

Instructions:

1. Place all of the ingredients in a blender and blend until smooth.

2. Pour into a glass and enjoy.

Ingredients:

- 2 tablespoons olive oil

- 2 cups diced sweet potatoes

- ½ cup chopped onion

- ¼ teaspoon ground cumin

- ¼ teaspoon ground coriander

- ½ teaspoon salt

- ¼ teaspoon black pepper

- 2 tablespoons chopped fresh parsley (optional)

Instructions:

1. Heat the olive oil in a large skillet over medium heat.

2. Add the sweet potatoes and onion, and cook for 10 minutes, stirring occasionally.

3. Add the cumin, coriander, salt, and pepper, and cook for an additional 10 minutes, stirring occasionally.

4. Serve in a bowl and top with fresh parsley, if desired.

Ingredients:

- 1 cup gluten-free all-purpose flour

- 1 teaspoon baking powder

- ¼ teaspoon salt

- 1 tablespoon sugar

- 1 cup almond milk

- 2 tablespoons melted coconut oil

- 1 teaspoon pure vanilla extract

Instructions:

1. Preheat a waffle iron according to the manufacturer's instructions.

2. In a medium bowl, whisk together the flour, baking powder, salt, and sugar.

3. In a separate bowl, whisk together the almond milk, coconut oil, and vanilla extract.

4. Pour the wet ingredients into the dry ingredients and whisk until just combined.

5. Pour the batter into the preheated waffle iron and cook according to the manufacturer's instructions.

Ingredients:

- 1 cup gluten-free all-purpose flour

- 1 teaspoon baking powder

- ½ teaspoon ground cinnamon

- 1 cup almond milk

- 2 tablespoons melted coconut oil

- 1 teaspoon pure vanilla extract

- 1 medium apple, peeled and grated

Instructions:

1. In a medium bowl, whisk together the flour, baking powder, and cinnamon.

2. In a separate bowl, whisk together the almond milk, coconut oil, and vanilla extract.

3. Pour the wet ingredients into the dry ingredients and stir until just combined.

4. Fold in the grated apple.

5. Heat a large non-stick skillet over medium heat.

6. Pour ¼ cup of batter into the pan for each pancake.

7. Cook for 2-3 minutes, or until the edges are golden brown.

8. Flip and cook for an additional 2-3 minutes, or until cooked through.

9. Serve hot.

Ingredients:

- 3 cups gluten-free rolled oats

- 1 cup chopped nuts (e.g., almonds, walnuts, pecans)

- ¼ cup honey

- 2 tablespoons melted coconut oil

- 1 teaspoon ground cinnamon

- ¼ teaspoon ground nutmeg

- ½ cup dried fruit (e.g., raisins, cranberries, apricots)

Instructions:

1. Preheat the oven to 350°F.

2. In a large bowl, combine the oats, nuts, honey, coconut oil, cinnamon, and nutmeg.

3. Spread the mixture onto a baking sheet and bake for 15-20 minutes, stirring once or twice during baking.

4. Remove from the oven and let cool.

5. Once cool, stir in the dried fruit.

6. Store in an airtight container.

Ingredients:

- 2 tablespoons olive oil

- ½ cup chopped onion

- ½ cup chopped bell pepper

- ½ cup chopped mushrooms

- 4 large eggs

- Salt and pepper to taste

Instructions:

1. Preheat the oven to 375°F.

2. Heat the olive oil in a large oven-safe skillet over medium heat.

3. Add the onion, bell pepper, and mushrooms, and cook for 5 minutes, stirring occasionally.

4. Crack the eggs into the skillet and season with salt and pepper.

5. Transfer the skillet to the oven and bake for 15-20 minutes, or until the eggs are cooked to your desired doneness.

6. Serve hot.

1. Baked Apple Slices with Walnuts (10 minutes)

Ingredients:

- 2 apples

- 2 tablespoons of chopped walnuts

- 2 tablespoons of honey

- Ground cinnamon

Instructions:

1. Preheat oven to 350°F.

2. Slice the apples into thin slices and place them on a baking sheet.

3. Sprinkle the walnuts over the apples and drizzle honey over them.

4. Sprinkle with ground cinnamon.

5. Bake for 10 minutes or until the apples are softened.

Ingredients:

- 1/2 cup of gluten-free pretzels

- 1/4 cup of dried cranberries

- 1/4 cup of roasted sunflower seeds

- 2 tablespoons of dark chocolate chips

Instructions:

1. In a bowl, mix the pretzels, cranberries, sunflower seeds and dark chocolate chips.

2. Spread the mixture on a baking sheet.

3. Bake at 350°F for 10 minutes or until lightly toasted.

Ingredients:

- 3 tablespoons of butter

- 1/4 cup of honey

- 1/4 cup of light corn syrup

- 4 cups of air-popped popcorn

Instructions:

1. In a medium saucepan, melt butter over low heat.

2. Add honey and corn syrup and stir until combined.

3. Pour the syrup mixture over the popcorn and stir until combined.

4. Scoop the popcorn mixture into balls and place them on a baking sheet lined with parchment paper.

5. Place the baking sheet in the refrigerator to chill for 30 minutes.

Ingredients:

- 2 ripe bananas

- 2 tablespoons of melted coconut oil

- Ground cinnamon

Instructions:

1. Preheat oven to 375°F.

2. Slice the bananas into thin slices and place them on a baking sheet.

3. Drizzle the melted coconut oil over the slices.

4. Sprinkle with ground cinnamon.

5. Bake for 25 minutes or until the chips are golden and crisp.

Ingredients:

- 1/2 cup of gluten-free oats

- 1/4 cup of shredded coconut

- 1/4 cup of almond butter

- 2 tablespoons of honey

- 2 tablespoons of chopped almonds

Instructions:

1. Preheat oven to 350°F.

2. In a bowl, mix the oats, coconut, almond butter and honey until combined.

3. Spread the mixture onto a baking sheet lined with parchment paper.

4. Sprinkle with chopped almonds.

5. Bake for 20 minutes or until golden brown.

Ingredients:

- 2 cups of grated zucchini

- 1/4 cup of gluten-free flour

- 1/4 cup of shredded Parmesan cheese

- 2 tablespoons of olive oil

- Ground black pepper

Instructions:

1. In a bowl, mix the zucchini, flour, Parmesan cheese and black pepper.

2. Heat the olive oil in a large skillet over medium heat.

3. Scoop the zucchini mixture into the skillet and flatten into fritters.

4. Cook for about 10 minutes on each side or until golden brown.

Ingredients:

- 1/2 cup of cubed cantaloupe

- 1/2 cup of cubed honeydew melon

- 1/2 cup of cubed pineapple

- 1/4 cup of sliced strawberries

- 2 tablespoons of honey

Instructions:

1. In a bowl, mix the cantaloupe, honeydew, pineapple and strawberries.

2. Drizzle the honey over the fruit salad and stir until combined.

3. Refrigerate for 15 minutes before serving.

Ingredients:

- 1/2 cup of gluten-free pizza sauce

- 1/2 cup of shredded mozzarella cheese

- 1/4 cup of diced bell peppers

- 2 tablespoons of chopped olives

- 2 gluten-free pizza crusts

Instructions:

1. Preheat oven to 375°F.

2. Spread the pizza sauce over the pizza crusts.

3. Top the crusts with cheese, bell peppers, and olives.

4. Bake for 20 minutes or until the cheese is melted and bubbly.

Ingredients:

- 1/2 cup of chopped dark chocolate

- 1/4 cup of chopped almonds

- 1/4 cup of chopped dried cranberries

Instructions:

1. Line a baking sheet with parchment paper.

2. Melt the dark chocolate in a double boiler over low heat.

3. Spread the melted chocolate onto the parchment paper.

4. Sprinkle with almonds and cranberries.

5. Refrigerate for 15 minutes or until the chocolate is set.

Ingredients:

- 1/2 cup of almonds

- 1/2 cup of walnuts

- 2 tablespoons of honey

- 1/4 teaspoon of ground cinnamon

Instructions:

1. Preheat oven to 375°F.

2. Spread the almonds and walnuts onto a baking sheet.

3. Drizzle the honey over the nuts and sprinkle with cinnamon.

4. Bake for 20 minutes or until golden brown.

6.3 LUNCH RECIPES

1. Tomato and Mozzarella Salad (15 minutes)

Ingredients:

-2 large tomatoes, sliced

-1/2 cup sliced mozzarella cheese

-2 tablespoons extra-virgin olive oil

-1 tablespoon balsamic vinegar

-salt and pepper, to taste

Instructions:

1. Slice tomatoes and mozzarella cheese and place in a bowl.

2. Drizzle with extra-virgin olive oil and balsamic vinegar.

3. Season with salt and pepper, to taste.

4. Serve and enjoy.

Ingredients:

-1/2 pound boneless, skinless chicken breasts

-1 tablespoon olive oil

-1/2 teaspoon garlic powder

-1/2 teaspoon onion powder

-1/2 teaspoon dried oregano

-salt and pepper, to taste

-1 bell pepper, sliced

-1 onion, sliced

Instructions:

1. Preheat the grill to medium heat.

2. Rub chicken breasts with olive oil, garlic powder, onion powder, dried oregano, salt, and pepper.

3. Place chicken and vegetables on the grill and cook for 10 minutes. Flip chicken and vegetables and continue cooking for an additional 5-10 minutes, or until chicken is cooked through and vegetables are tender.

4. Serve and enjoy.

Ingredients:

-1 large eggplant, cut into cubes

-1 large tomato, cut into cubes

-2 tablespoons olive oil

-1 teaspoon dried oregano

-1/2 teaspoon garlic powder

-salt and pepper, to taste

Instructions:

1. Preheat oven to 400°F.

2. Place eggplant and tomato cubes on a baking sheet.

3. Drizzle with olive oil and sprinkle with oregano, garlic powder, salt, and pepper.

4. Roast for 20 minutes, or until vegetables are tender and lightly browned.

5. Serve and enjoy.

Ingredients:

-1 cup cooked quinoa

-1/2 cup chopped broccoli

-1/2 cup chopped carrots

-1/2 cup chopped bell pepper

-2 tablespoons olive oil

-1 teaspoon garlic powder

-1 teaspoon dried oregano

-salt and pepper, to taste

Instructions:

1. In a large bowl, combine cooked quinoa, broccoli, carrots, and bell pepper.

2. Drizzle with olive oil and sprinkle with garlic powder, oregano, salt, and pepper.

3. Toss to combine.

4. Heat a large skillet over medium heat.

5. Add quinoa and vegetable mixture and cook for 10 minutes, stirring occasionally.

6. Serve and enjoy.

Ingredients:

-4 ounces cooked salmon

-2 cups spinach leaves

-1/4 cup sliced red onion

-1/4 cup sliced cucumber

-1/4 cup crumbled feta cheese

-2 tablespoons olive oil

-1 tablespoon lemon juice

-salt and pepper, to taste

Instructions:

1. Place spinach leaves in a bowl.

2. Top with salmon, red onion, cucumber, and feta cheese.

3. Drizzle with olive oil and lemon juice.

4. Season with salt and pepper, to taste.

5. Serve and enjoy.

Ingredients:

-2 slices gluten-free bread

-2 slices turkey

-1/4 avocado, mashed

-1 tablespoon mayonnaise

-1/4 teaspoon garlic powder

-salt and pepper, to taste

Instructions:

1. Toast slices of gluten-free bread.

2. Spread mashed avocado on one slice of toast and mayonnaise on the other slice.

3. Sprinkle garlic powder, salt, and pepper on the avocado.

4. Top with turkey slices.

5. Place the other slice of toast on top and cut in half.

6. Serve and enjoy.

Ingredients:

-2 zucchinis, spiralized

-1/2 cup cherry tomatoes, halved

-1/4 cup chopped olives

-1 tablespoon olive oil

-1/2 teaspoon garlic powder

-salt and pepper, to taste

Instructions:

1. Heat a large skillet over medium heat.

2. Add spiralized zucchini noodles and cook for 5 minutes.

3. Add cherry tomatoes and olives and cook for an additional 5 minutes.

4. Drizzle with olive oil and sprinkle with garlic powder, salt, and pepper.

5. Toss to combine.

6. Serve and enjoy.

Ingredients:

-2 gluten-free tortillas

-4 ounces canned tuna, drained

-1/4 cup diced tomatoes

-1/4 cup diced cucumbers

-1/4 cup crumbled feta cheese

-2 tablespoons olive oil

-1 tablespoon lemon juice

-salt and pepper, to taste

Instructions:

1. Spread tuna onto gluten-free tortillas.

2. Top with tomatoes, cucumbers, and feta cheese.

3. Drizzle with olive oil and lemon juice.

4. Season with salt and pepper, to taste.

5. Roll up and serve.

Ingredients:

-1 package frozen spinach, thawed and drained

-1 can artichoke hearts, drained and chopped

-1/2 cup grated parmesan cheese

-1/2 cup mayonnaise

-1/2 teaspoon garlic powder

-salt and pepper, to taste

Instructions:

1. Preheat oven to 350°F.

2. In a bowl, combine spinach, artichoke hearts, parmesan cheese, mayonnaise, garlic powder, salt, and pepper.

3. Spread mixture into a baking dish.

4. Bake for 20 minutes.

5. Serve with gluten-free crackers or chips.

Ingredients:

-2 large sweet potatoes, cut into wedges

-2 tablespoons olive oil

-1 teaspoon garlic powder

-1 teaspoon dried oregano

-salt and pepper, to taste

Instructions:

1. Preheat oven to 400°F.

2. Place sweet potato wedges on a baking sheet.

3. Drizzle with olive oil and sprinkle with garlic powder, oregano, salt, and pepper.

4. Roast for 25 minutes, or until potatoes are tender and lightly browned.

5. Serve and enjoy.

1. Baked Salmon with Quinoa Pilaf (30 minutes)

Ingredients:

-1/2 cup quinoa

-1/2 cup water

-1/4 cup diced onion

-1/4 cup diced carrots

-1/4 cup diced celery

-2 cloves garlic, minced

-1 tablespoon olive oil

-2 tablespoons lemon juice

-1/4 teaspoon dried oregano

-1/4 teaspoon dried thyme

-1/4 teaspoon sea salt

-4 ounces wild-caught salmon

Instructions:

1. Preheat oven to 375°F and line a baking sheet with parchment paper.

2. In a small saucepan, add quinoa and water and bring to a boil. Reduce heat, cover and simmer for 15 minutes, or until quinoa is cooked.

3. In a medium skillet, add onion, carrots, celery, garlic, olive oil, lemon juice, oregano, thyme and sea salt. Cook over medium heat for 8-10 minutes, stirring occasionally.

4. Stir in cooked quinoa and transfer to the prepared baking sheet.

5. Place salmon on top of quinoa pilaf and bake for 15 minutes, or until salmon is cooked through.

Ingredients:

-1 large onion, diced

-4 cloves garlic, minced

-2 carrots, diced

-2 celery stalks, diced

-2 potatoes, diced

-1/4 teaspoon sea salt

-1/4 teaspoon black pepper

-1 teaspoon dried oregano

-1 teaspoon dried basil

-1 teaspoon dried thyme

-1/2 teaspoon paprika

-1/2 teaspoon garlic powder

-1/2 teaspoon onion powder

-1/2 teaspoon chili powder

-3 cups vegetable broth

-1 (14.5 ounce) can diced tomatoes

Instructions:

1. Preheat oven to 375°F and line a baking sheet with parchment paper.

2. Add onion, garlic, carrots, celery, potatoes, sea salt, black pepper, oregano, basil, thyme, paprika, garlic powder, onion powder, and chili powder to the baking sheet. Toss to combine.

3. Roast vegetables in preheated oven for 25 minutes, stirring once halfway through.

4. Meanwhile, add vegetable broth and diced tomatoes to a large pot and bring to a boil over medium-high heat.

5. Reduce heat to low and add roasted vegetables to the pot. Simmer for 20 minutes.

6. Serve warm.

Ingredients:

-1 pound boneless, skinless chicken breasts

-1/2 cup white rice

-1/2 cup diced onion

-1 cup diced carrots

-1 cup diced celery

-1/2 teaspoon sea salt

-1/2 teaspoon black pepper

-1 teaspoon garlic powder

-1 teaspoon onion powder

-1/2 teaspoon dried oregano

-1/2 teaspoon dried thyme

-1/4 teaspoon dried basil

-4 cups chicken broth

Instructions:

1. Add chicken breasts, rice, onion, carrots, celery, sea salt, black pepper, garlic powder, onion powder, oregano, thyme, and basil to a slow cooker.

2. Pour chicken broth over the top and stir to combine.

3. Cook on low for 6 hours or until chicken is cooked through and rice is tender.

4. Serve warm.

Ingredients:

-1/2 cup quinoa

-1 cup water

-1 tablespoon olive oil

-1/2 cup diced onion

-1 cup diced carrots

-1 cup diced celery

-1/2 teaspoon sea salt

-1/2 teaspoon black pepper

-2 cloves garlic, minced

-1 tablespoon freshly grated ginger

-2 tablespoons tamari

-2 tablespoons freshly squeezed lemon juice

Instructions:

1. In a small saucepan, add quinoa and water and bring to a boil. Reduce heat, cover and simmer for 15 minutes, or until quinoa is cooked.

2. Heat olive oil in a large skillet over medium-high heat.

3. Add onion, carrots, celery, sea salt, black pepper, garlic, and ginger to the skillet and cook for 5 minutes, stirring occasionally.

4. Reduce heat to low and add cooked quinoa, tamari, and lemon juice. Stir to combine.

5. Cook for an additional 5 minutes, stirring occasionally.

6. Serve warm.

Ingredients:

-1 pound Brussels sprouts, trimmed and halved

-1 tablespoon olive oil

-1/2 teaspoon sea salt

-1/4 teaspoon black pepper

-2 cloves garlic, minced

-1/2 teaspoon dried oregano

-1/2 teaspoon dried thyme

-1/4 teaspoon dried basil

-1 (14 ounce) package extra-firm tofu, drained and cubed

-2 tablespoons tamari

Instructions:

1. Preheat oven to 375°F and line a baking sheet with parchment paper.

2. Add Brussels sprouts, olive oil, sea salt, black pepper, garlic, oregano, thyme, and basil to the prepared baking sheet. Toss to combine.

3. Bake in preheated oven for 20 minutes, stirring once halfway through.

4. Meanwhile, add tofu cubes to a bowl and toss with tamari.

5. Add tofu to the baking sheet with the Brussels sprouts and continue baking for an additional 10 minutes, stirring once.

6. Serve warm.

Ingredients:

-1/2 cup quinoa

-1 cup water

-1 tablespoon olive oil

-1/2 cup diced onion

-1 cup diced carrots

-1 cup diced celery

-1/2 teaspoon sea salt

-1/2 teaspoon black pepper

-2 cloves garlic, minced

-1/2 teaspoon dried oregano

-1/2 teaspoon dried thyme

-1/4 teaspoon dried basil

-1 (14.5 ounce) can diced tomatoes

Instructions:

1. In a small saucepan, add quinoa and water and bring to a boil. Reduce heat, cover and simmer for 15 minutes, or until quinoa is cooked.

2. Heat olive oil in a large skillet over medium-high heat.

3. Add onion, carrots, celery, sea salt, black pepper, garlic, oregano, thyme, and basil. Cook for 5 minutes, stirring occasionally.

4. Reduce heat to low and add cooked quinoa and diced tomatoes. Stir to combine.

5. Cook for an additional 5 minutes, stirring occasionally.

6. Serve warm.

Ingredients:

-2 boneless, skinless chicken breasts

-1/2 teaspoon sea salt

-1/4 teaspoon black pepper

-2 tablespoons olive oil

-1/2 teaspoon garlic powder

-1/2 teaspoon onion powder

-1/2 teaspoon dried oregano

-1/2 teaspoon dried thyme

-2 zucchini, sliced

Instructions:

1. Preheat grill to medium-high heat.

2. Season chicken breasts with sea salt, black pepper, olive oil, garlic powder, onion powder, oregano, and thyme.

3. Grill chicken for 10 minutes, flipping once, or until chicken is cooked through.

4. Add zucchini slices to the grill and cook for 5 minutes, flipping once.

5. Serve chicken and zucchini warm.

Ingredients:

-2 sweet potatoes, cubed

-1 tablespoon olive oil

-1/2 teaspoon sea salt

-1/4 teaspoon black pepper

-1/2 teaspoon garlic powder

-1/2 teaspoon onion powder

-1/2 teaspoon dried oregano

-1/2 teaspoon dried thyme

-1 cup broccoli florets

Instructions:

1. Preheat oven to 375°F and line a baking sheet with parchment paper.

2. Add sweet potatoes, olive oil, sea salt, black pepper, garlic powder, onion powder, oregano, and thyme to the prepared baking sheet. Toss to combine.

3. Bake in preheated oven for 20 minutes, stirring once halfway through.

4. Add broccoli florets to the baking sheet with the sweet potatoes and continue baking for an additional 15 minutes, stirring once.

5. Serve warm.

Ingredients:

-1 large onion, diced

-4 cloves garlic, minced

-2 carrots, diced

-2 celery stalks, diced

-2 potatoes, diced

-1/4 teaspoon sea salt

-1/4 teaspoon black pepper

-1 teaspoon dried oregano

-1 teaspoon dried basil

-1 teaspoon dried thyme

-1/2 teaspoon paprika

-1/2 teaspoon garlic powder

-1/2 teaspoon onion powder

-1/2 teaspoon chili powder

-3 cups vegetable broth

-1 (14.5 ounce) can diced tomatoes

Instructions:

1. Add onion, garlic, carrots, celery, potatoes, sea salt, black pepper, oregano, basil, thyme, paprika, garlic powder, onion powder, and chili powder to a slow cooker.

2. Pour vegetable broth and diced tomatoes over the top and stir to combine.

3. Cook on low for 6 hours or until vegetables are tender.

4. Serve warm.

Ingredients:

-1 tablespoon olive oil

-1/2 cup diced onion

-1 tablespoon freshly grated ginger

-2 cloves garlic, minced

-1 teaspoon ground cumin

-1 teaspoon ground coriander

-1/2 teaspoon sea salt

-1/4 teaspoon black pepper

-1 teaspoon curry powder

-1 (14.5 ounce) can diced tomatoes

-1 cup dried green lentils

-3 cups vegetable broth

-1/2 cup coconut milk

Instructions:

1. Heat olive oil in a large pot over medium-high heat.

2. Add onion, ginger, garlic, cumin, coriander, sea salt, black pepper, and curry powder. Cook for 3 minutes, stirring often.

3. Add diced tomatoes, lentils, and vegetable broth. Bring to a boil, reduce heat, cover and simmer for 30 minutes, or until lentils are tender.

4. Stir in coconut milk and cook for an additional 5 minutes.

5. Serve warm.

6.5 DESSERT RECIPES

1. Gluten-Free Apple Crisp (45 minutes)

Ingredients:

-3 large apples, peeled and thinly sliced

-1/2 cup gluten-free oats

-1/2 cup gluten-free flour

-1/2 cup packed brown sugar

-1 teaspoon ground cinnamon

-1/4 teaspoon salt

-1/4 cup cold butter

Instructions:

1. Preheat oven to 350°F.

2. Place the sliced apples in an 8x8-inch baking dish.

3. In a medium bowl, mix together oats, flour, brown sugar, cinnamon, and salt.

4. Cut the butter into the dry ingredients until it resembles coarse crumbs.

5. Sprinkle the crumb mixture over the apples.

6. Bake for 45 minutes or until the top is golden brown and the apples are tender.

7. Serve warm.

Ingredients:

-3 tablespoons cornstarch

-2/3 cup granulated sugar

-1/4 teaspoon salt

-2 cups milk

-2 ounces semi-sweet chocolate, chopped

-1 teaspoon pure vanilla extract

Instructions:

1. In a medium saucepan, whisk together the cornstarch, sugar, and salt.

2. Gradually whisk in the milk.

3. Place over medium heat and cook, stirring constantly, until the mixture comes to a boil.

4. Reduce the heat to low and continue to cook, stirring constantly, for 2 minutes.

5. Remove from the heat and stir in the chopped chocolate and vanilla extract.

6. Pour the pudding into individual serving dishes.

7. Place plastic wrap directly onto the surface of the pudding.

8. Place in the refrigerator to chill for 30 minutes.

9. Serve chilled.

Ingredients:

-1 gluten-free pie crust

-6 cups fresh or frozen blueberries

-1/2 cup granulated sugar

-1/4 cup cornstarch

-1/4 teaspoon ground cinnamon

-1/8 teaspoon salt

Instructions:

1. Preheat oven to 375°F.

2. Place the pie crust in a 9-inch pie plate.

3. In a large bowl, mix together the blueberries, sugar, cornstarch, cinnamon, and salt.

4. Pour the berry mixture into the pie crust.

5. Bake for 50 minutes or until the filling is bubbly and the crust is golden brown.

6. Let cool for 20 minutes before serving.

Ingredients:

-2 cups shredded coconut

-1/2 cup granulated sugar

-1/4 teaspoon salt

-2 large egg whites

-1 teaspoon pure vanilla extract

Instructions:

1. Preheat oven to 350°F.

2. Line a baking sheet with parchment paper.

3. In a medium bowl, mix together the shredded coconut, sugar, and salt.

4. In a separate bowl, whisk together the egg whites and vanilla extract.

5. Pour the egg mixture into the coconut mixture and stir until well combined.

6. Using a spoon, drop the batter onto the prepared baking sheet.

7. Bake for 25 minutes or until golden brown.

8. Let cool before serving.

Ingredients:

-2 cups gluten-free flour

-1 teaspoon baking soda

-1/4 teaspoon salt

-1/2 cup vegetable oil

-3/4 cup packed brown sugar

-2 large eggs

-3 ripe bananas, mashed

Instructions:

1. Preheat oven to 350°F.

2. Grease a 9x5-inch loaf pan.

3. In a large bowl, whisk together flour, baking soda, and salt.

4. In a separate bowl, mix together oil, sugar, eggs, and mashed bananas.

5. Pour the wet ingredients into the dry ingredients and stir until well combined.

6. Pour the batter into the prepared loaf pan.

7. Bake for 60 minutes or until a toothpick inserted into the center comes out clean.

8. Let cool for 10 minutes before serving.

Ingredients:

-3/4 cup gluten-free flour

-1/2 teaspoon baking soda

-1/4 teaspoon salt

-1/2 cup butter, softened

-1/2 cup packed brown sugar

-1/4 cup granulated sugar

-1 large egg

-1 teaspoon pure vanilla extract

-1 cup semi-sweet chocolate chips

Instructions:

1. Preheat oven to 375°F.

2. Line a baking sheet with parchment paper.

3. In a medium bowl, whisk together the flour, baking soda, and salt.

4. In a separate bowl, cream together the butter and sugars until light and fluffy.

5. Add the egg and vanilla extract and mix until combined.

6. Gradually add the dry ingredients to the wet ingredients and mix until well combined.

7. Stir in the chocolate chips.

8. Using a spoon, drop the batter onto the prepared baking sheet.

9. Bake for 15 minutes or until golden brown.

10. Let cool before serving.

Ingredients:

-2 cups gluten-free flour

-2 teaspoons baking powder

-1 teaspoon baking soda

-1/2 teaspoon salt

-2 teaspoons ground cinnamon

-1/2 cup vegetable oil

-1 cup packed brown sugar

-3 large eggs

-2 cups grated carrots

-1/2 cup raisins

Instructions:

1. Preheat oven to 350°F.

2. Grease a 9x13-inch baking pan.

3. In a large bowl, whisk together the flour, baking powder, baking soda, salt, and cinnamon.

4. In a separate bowl, mix together the oil, sugar, and eggs.

5. Pour the wet ingredients into the dry ingredients and stir until well combined.

6. Stir in the carrots and raisins.

7. Pour the batter into the prepared baking pan.

8. Bake for 1 hour or until a toothpick inserted into the center comes out clean.

9. Let cool for 10 minutes before serving.

Ingredients:

-3/4 cup gluten-free flour

-1/2 teaspoon baking powder

-1/4 teaspoon salt

-1/2 cup butter, softened

-1 cup granulated sugar

-3 large eggs

-1 teaspoon pure vanilla extract

Instructions:

1. Preheat oven to 350°F.

2. Grease a 9x5-inch loaf pan.

3. In a medium bowl, whisk together the flour, baking powder, and salt.

4. In a separate bowl, cream together the butter and sugar until light and fluffy.

5. Add the eggs one at a time, mixing well after each addition.

6. Add the vanilla extract.

7. Gradually add the dry ingredients to the wet ingredients and mix until well combined.

8. Pour the batter into the prepared loaf pan.

9. Bake for 1 hour or until a toothpick inserted into the center comes out clean.

10. Let cool for 10 minutes before serving.

Ingredients:

-4 cups sliced fresh peaches

-1/2 cup granulated sugar

-1/4 cup cornstarch

-1/2 teaspoon ground cinnamon

-1/8 teaspoon salt

-1/2 cup gluten-free flour

-1/2 cup packed brown sugar

-1/4 cup cold butter

Instructions:

1. Preheat oven to 375°F.

2. Grease a 9x9-inch baking dish.

3. In a large bowl, mix together the peaches, sugar, cornstarch, cinnamon, and salt.

4. Pour the peach mixture into the prepared baking dish.

5. In a medium bowl, mix together the flour and brown sugar.

6. Cut the butter into the dry ingredients until it resembles coarse crumbs.

7. Sprinkle the crumb mixture over the peaches.

8. Bake for 45 minutes or until the top is golden brown and the peaches are tender.

9. Let cool for 15 minutes before serving.

Ingredients:

-2 cups diced fresh pineapple

-2 cups diced fresh strawberries

-1 cup diced fresh mango

-1/2 cup diced fresh kiwi

-1/2 cup diced fresh papaya

-1/4 cup honey

-1 teaspoon freshly squeezed lemon juice

Instructions:

1. In a large bowl, mix together the pineapple, strawberries, mango, kiwi, and papaya.

2. In a small bowl, mix together the honey and lemon juice until well combined.

3. Pour the honey mixture over the fruit and stir until evenly coated.

4. Serve chilled.

Weekly Meal Planner

Week................

	BREAKFAST	LUNCH	DINNER	SNACKS
MON				
TUE				
WED				
THU				
FRI				
SAT				
SUN				

Grocery List :

Weekly Meal Planner

Week................

	BREAKFAST	LUNCH	DINNER	SNACKS
MON				
TUE				
WED				
THU				
FRI				
SAT				
SUN				

Grocery List :

Weekly Meal Planner

Week................

	BREAKFAST	LUNCH	DINNER	SNACKS
MON				
TUE				
WED				
THU				
FRI				
SAT				
SUN				

Grocery List :

Weekly Meal Planner

Week................

	BREAKFAST	LUNCH	DINNER	SNACKS
MON				
TUE				
WED				
THU				
FRI				
SAT				
SUN				

Grocery List :

Weekly Meal Planner

Week................

	BREAKFAST	LUNCH	DINNER	SNACKS
MON				
TUE				
WED				
THU				
FRI				
SAT				
SUN				

Grocery List :

Weekly Meal Planner

Week...............

	BREAKFAST	LUNCH	DINNER	SNACKS
MON				
TUE				
WED				
THU				
FRI				
SAT				
SUN				

Grocery List :

Weekly Meal Planner

Week................

	BREAKFAST	LUNCH	DINNER	SNACKS
MON				
TUE				
WED				
THU				
FRI				
SAT				
SUN				

Grocery List :

___________________ ___________________ ___________________
___________________ ___________________ ___________________
___________________ ___________________ ___________________
___________________ ___________________ ___________________
___________________ ___________________ ___________________
___________________ ___________________ ___________________

Weekly Meal Planner

Week................

	BREAKFAST	LUNCH	DINNER	SNACKS
MON				
TUE				
WED				
THU				
FRI				
SAT				
SUN				

Grocery List :

Weekly Meal Planner

Week................

	BREAKFAST	LUNCH	DINNER	SNACKS
MON				
TUE				
WED				
THU				
FRI				
SAT				
SUN				

Grocery List :

Weekly Meal Planner

Week................

	BREAKFAST	LUNCH	DINNER	SNACKS
MON				
TUE				
WED				
THU				
FRI				
SAT				
SUN				

Grocery List :

______________ ______________ ______________
______________ ______________ ______________
______________ ______________ ______________
______________ ______________ ______________
______________ ______________ ______________
______________ ______________ ______________

Weekly Meal Planner

Week................

	BREAKFAST	LUNCH	DINNER	SNACKS
MON				
TUE				
WED				
THU				
FRI				
SAT				
SUN				

Grocery List :

Weekly Meal Planner

Week................

	BREAKFAST	LUNCH	DINNER	SNACKS
MON				
TUE				
WED				
THU				
FRI				
SAT				
SUN				

Grocery List :

Weekly Meal Planner

Week................

	BREAKFAST	LUNCH	DINNER	SNACKS
MON				
TUE				
WED				
THU				
FRI				
SAT				
SUN				

Grocery List :

Weekly Meal Planner

Week................

	BREAKFAST	LUNCH	DINNER	SNACKS
MON				
TUE				
WED				
THU				
FRI				
SAT				
SUN				

Grocery List :

Weekly Meal Planner

Week.................

	BREAKFAST	LUNCH	DINNER	SNACKS
MON				
TUE				
WED				
THU				
FRI				
SAT				
SUN				

Grocery List :

Weekly Meal Planner

Week...............

	BREAKFAST	LUNCH	DINNER	SNACKS
MON				
TUE				
WED				
THU				
FRI				
SAT				
SUN				

Grocery List :
_____________ _____________ _____________
_____________ _____________ _____________
_____________ _____________ _____________
_____________ _____________ _____________
_____________ _____________ _____________
_____________ _____________ _____________

Weekly Meal Planner

Week................

	BREAKFAST	LUNCH	DINNER	SNACKS
MON				
TUE				
WED				
THU				
FRI				
SAT				
SUN				

Grocery List :

Weekly Meal Planner

Week................

	BREAKFAST	LUNCH	DINNER	SNACKS
MON				
TUE				
WED				
THU				
FRI				
SAT				
SUN				

Grocery List :
_____________________ _____________________ _____________________
_____________________ _____________________ _____________________
_____________________ _____________________ _____________________
_____________________ _____________________ _____________________
_____________________ _____________________ _____________________

Weekly Meal Planner

Week................

	BREAKFAST	LUNCH	DINNER	SNACKS
MON				
TUE				
WED				
THU				
FRI				
SAT				
SUN				

Grocery List :

Weekly Meal Planner

Week................

	BREAKFAST	LUNCH	DINNER	SNACKS
MON				
TUE				
WED				
THU				
FRI				
SAT				
SUN				

Grocery List :

Weekly Meal Planner

Week................

	BREAKFAST	LUNCH	DINNER	SNACKS
MON				
TUE				
WED				
THU				
FRI				
SAT				
SUN				

Grocery List :

Weekly Meal Planner

Week...............

	BREAKFAST	LUNCH	DINNER	SNACKS
MON				
TUE				
WED				
THU				
FRI				
SAT				
SUN				

Grocery List :

Weekly Meal Planner

Week................

	BREAKFAST	LUNCH	DINNER	SNACKS
MON				
TUE				
WED				
THU				
FRI				
SAT				
SUN				

Grocery List :
_______________ _______________ _______________
_______________ _______________ _______________
_______________ _______________ _______________
_______________ _______________ _______________
_______________ _______________ _______________

Weekly Meal Planner

Week................

	BREAKFAST	LUNCH	DINNER	SNACKS
MON				
TUE				
WED				
THU				
FRI				
SAT				
SUN				

Grocery List :

_________________ _________________ _________________
_________________ _________________ _________________
_________________ _________________ _________________
_________________ _________________ _________________
_________________ _________________ _________________

Weekly Meal Planner

Week................

	BREAKFAST	LUNCH	DINNER	SNACKS
MON				
TUE				
WED				
THU				
FRI				
SAT				
SUN				

Grocery List :

Weekly Meal Planner

Week................

	BREAKFAST	LUNCH	DINNER	SNACKS
MON				
TUE				
WED				
THU				
FRI				
SAT				
SUN				

Grocery List :

Weekly Meal Planner

Week................

	BREAKFAST	LUNCH	DINNER	SNACKS
MON				
TUE				
WED				
THU				
FRI				
SAT				
SUN				

Grocery List :

Weekly Meal Planner

Week................

	BREAKFAST	LUNCH	DINNER	SNACKS
MON				
TUE				
WED				
THU				
FRI				
SAT				
SUN				

Grocery List :

Weekly Meal Planner

Week.................

	BREAKFAST	LUNCH	DINNER	SNACKS
MON				
TUE				
WED				
THU				
FRI				
SAT				
SUN				

Grocery List :

Weekly Meal Planner

Week................

	BREAKFAST	LUNCH	DINNER	SNACKS
MON				
TUE				
WED				
THU				
FRI				
SAT				
SUN				

Grocery List :

Weekly Meal Planner

Week................

	BREAKFAST	LUNCH	DINNER	SNACKS
MON				
TUE				
WED				
THU				
FRI				
SAT				
SUN				

Grocery List :
_______________ _______________ _______________
_______________ _______________ _______________
_______________ _______________ _______________
_______________ _______________ _______________
_______________ _______________ _______________

Weekly Meal Planner

Week...............

	BREAKFAST	LUNCH	DINNER	SNACKS
MON				
TUE				
WED				
THU				
FRI				
SAT				
SUN				

Grocery List :

Weekly Meal Planner

Week................

	BREAKFAST	LUNCH	DINNER	SNACKS
MON				
TUE				
WED				
THU				
FRI				
SAT				
SUN				

Grocery List :

Weekly Meal Planner

Week................

	BREAKFAST	LUNCH	DINNER	SNACKS
MON				
TUE				
WED				
THU				
FRI				
SAT				
SUN				

Grocery List :
______________ ______________ ______________
______________ ______________ ______________
______________ ______________ ______________
______________ ______________ ______________
______________ ______________ ______________
______________ ______________ ______________

Weekly Meal Planner

Week................

	BREAKFAST	LUNCH	DINNER	SNACKS
MON				
TUE				
WED				
THU				
FRI				
SAT				
SUN				

Grocery List :

Weekly Meal Planner

Week................

	BREAKFAST	LUNCH	DINNER	SNACKS
MON				
TUE				
WED				
THU				
FRI				
SAT				
SUN				

Grocery List :

Weekly Meal Planner

Week................

	BREAKFAST	LUNCH	DINNER	SNACKS
MON				
TUE				
WED				
THU				
FRI				
SAT				
SUN				

Grocery List :

Weekly Meal Planner

Week................

	BREAKFAST	LUNCH	DINNER	SNACKS
MON				
TUE				
WED				
THU				
FRI				
SAT				
SUN				

Grocery List :

Weekly Meal Planner

Week................

	BREAKFAST	LUNCH	DINNER	SNACKS
MON				
TUE				
WED				
THU				
FRI				
SAT				
SUN				

Grocery List :

________________ ________________ ________________
________________ ________________ ________________
________________ ________________ ________________
________________ ________________ ________________
________________ ________________ ________________
________________ ________________ ________________

Weekly Meal Planner

Week................

	BREAKFAST	LUNCH	DINNER	SNACKS
MON				
TUE				
WED				
THU				
FRI				
SAT				
SUN				

Grocery List :

Weekly Meal Planner

Week................

	BREAKFAST	LUNCH	DINNER	SNACKS
MON				
TUE				
WED				
THU				
FRI				
SAT				
SUN				

Grocery List :

Weekly Meal Planner

Week................

	BREAKFAST	LUNCH	DINNER	SNACKS
MON				
TUE				
WED				
THU				
FRI				
SAT				
SUN				

Grocery List :

Weekly Meal Planner

Week................

	BREAKFAST	LUNCH	DINNER	SNACKS
MON				
TUE				
WED				
THU				
FRI				
SAT				
SUN				

Grocery List :
_______________ _______________ _______________
_______________ _______________ _______________
_______________ _______________ _______________
_______________ _______________ _______________
_______________ _______________ _______________

Weekly Meal Planner

Week................

	BREAKFAST	LUNCH	DINNER	SNACKS
MON				
TUE				
WED				
THU				
FRI				
SAT				
SUN				

Grocery List :

Weekly Meal Planner

Week................

	BREAKFAST	LUNCH	DINNER	SNACKS
MON				
TUE				
WED				
THU				
FRI				
SAT				
SUN				

Grocery List :

Weekly Meal Planner

Week................

	BREAKFAST	LUNCH	DINNER	SNACKS
MON				
TUE				
WED				
THU				
FRI				
SAT				
SUN				

Grocery List :

Weekly Meal Planner

Week.................

	BREAKFAST	LUNCH	DINNER	SNACKS
MON				
TUE				
WED				
THU				
FRI				
SAT				
SUN				

Grocery List :

Weekly Meal Planner

Week................

	BREAKFAST	LUNCH	DINNER	SNACKS
MON				
TUE				
WED				
THU				
FRI				
SAT				
SUN				

Grocery List :

Weekly Meal Planner

Week................

	BREAKFAST	LUNCH	DINNER	SNACKS
MON				
TUE				
WED				
THU				
FRI				
SAT				
SUN				

Grocery List :

Weekly Meal Planner

Week................

	BREAKFAST	LUNCH	DINNER	SNACKS
MON				
TUE				
WED				
THU				
FRI				
SAT				
SUN				

Grocery List :

Weekly Meal Planner

Week................

	BREAKFAST	LUNCH	DINNER	SNACKS
MON				
TUE				
WED				
THU				
FRI				
SAT				
SUN				

Grocery List :

Weekly Meal Planner

Week...............

	BREAKFAST	LUNCH	DINNER	SNACKS
MON				
TUE				
WED				
THU				
FRI				
SAT				
SUN				

Grocery List :